Reactive

Your 5 Step Recovery Plan

Allison Francis, MAT & Betty Johnson, MD (Ed.)

Contents

Introduction

I can't pinpoint exactly when I first had symptoms of reactive hypoglycemia, but I suspect it was when I was a child – forty years before my eventual diagnosis. I was a difficult child, to say the least. The "trick" I used to do that drove my mother crazy was to faint when I became too angry or upset; the "attention getter" as my mother used to call it. As a teenager, the world would swim around me and I would pass out frequently.

Doctors could find nothing wrong and told me it was likely because of a temporary drop in blood pressure. I fainted after blood tests, passed out in clubs (and not because of drugs or alcohol), collapsed in grocery stores. I resigned myself that passing out was just part of who I was and there was nothing I could do about it.

Of course, looking back, I can see the less-obvious symptoms and signs of reactive hypoglycemia. Before I passed out, my brain would fog. My palms would get cold, clammy and sweaty. I would feel sick to my stomach and – once I recovered from "fainting" (which actually turned out to be petit mal seizures), I would often throw up or have severe stomach problems.

The reason that I went undiagnosed for over forty years was likely because reactive hypoglycemia isn't something that conveniently shows up in a doctor's office. By the time I actually got to see a doctor, I felt perfectly fine. My fainting spells tended to happen late afternoon or late evening; a glass of orange juice always made me feel better, I never made the link between how ill I felt and low blood sugar. In fact, I wasn't even aware that blood sugar could cause so many problems. Diabetes does not run in my family, I have no risk factors for the disease and so the conversation never came up at doctor's appointments. Why would it? A thin, active, healthy woman with excellent blood work complaining about "feeling faint" sometimes. I'm sure if I had said the "key phrases" to my doctor – sweating hands and shaking two hours after eating – he might have ordered me a test for reactive hypoglycemia. But back then, I just didn't know what was going on. I just knew I felt ill, a lot. I was constantly hungry or sometimes sick to my stomach and I didn't want to eat at all. I had severe mood swings which I put down to the stress of work, bills, relationships or whatever was ailing me at the time.

My turning point was when I posted on a health discussion board about stress and depression. By chance, a fellow poster had diabetes and said she felt that her blood sugar swings were causing most of her stress and depression. I found a free blood sugar monitor deal online (I just Googled "free blood sugar monitor") and a few days later my monitor arrived in the mail. I waited until I felt ill (4 p.m. on a Tuesday afternoon) and tested my blood sugar. It was 49 mg/dL. To put that in context, the "normal" range for fasting blood sugar is about 70mg/dL to 120 mg/dl. At 49 mg/dL, that's when the brain starts to malfunction, causing a host of neurological symptoms from "brain fog" to mood swings.

Follow up testing with an endocrinologist confirmed the diagnosis, but it wasn't all good news. "I hate giving this diagnosis," he said, "because there's nothing I can do for you." Of course, he did offer *some* suggestions – small, frequent meals, avoid soda, eat healthful meals. But instead of getting better, I actually got *worse*! In 2010, my blood sugar dipped to 25mg/dL and I had my first grand mal seizure. A grand mal seizure is basically where you pass out and have violent muscle contractions. I wasn't aware of the seizure, but it scared the heck out of my boyfriend, who called 911. I woke up in a daze in the ambulance.

The seizure was the final straw. I knew I had to do something. I scoured discussion boards and reactive hypoglycemia sites and found little help.

Luckily, my job at a local university gave me access to online medical journals, which was at least a good starting point. I went to see *six* different endocrinologists until I found one who was familiar enough with reactive hypoglycemia that I felt he knew what he was talking about. He was an MD/PhD at a local teaching hospital. He told me that there's a fair amount of recent (in the last 10 years or so) research that has recognized reactive hypoglycemia as an actual disorder with actual causes. "Anyone who went to medical school before 2000 probably isn't aware of the research," he said. As a specialist in endocrinology *and* a professor at the medical school, it was his job to keep up with current research. Doctors in general practice or even those doctors who practice endocrinology aren't always aware of the latest research – it's their job to see patients, not teach or write papers. My visit with this one endocrinologist was more insightful than all of my prior doctor's visits combined (30+ years of appointments!). So much so, that I would encourage you to seek out an endocrinologist at a local teaching hospital rather than seeing your local doctor. Reactive hypoglycemia is such a complex disease, and such a *miserable* disease, that it's worth the road trip if you don't have a teaching hospital in your area.

I also found a nutritionist who was familiar with the condition and he helped me tailor my diet. Finally, a good friend of mine who is a holistic physical therapist helped me tailor my exercise routine so that it didn't end up with me exercising too hard and dumping my blood sugar. The advice for many pre-diabetics, or anyone else with reactive hypoglycemia, is to lose weight and exercise. But what you might not realize is that too much exercise can also dump your blood sugar. The key is to finding that "sweet spot" – an exercise plan that will fit in with your goal of blood sugar stability.

The entire process, from that first grand mal seizure to feeling 100% took about three years, mostly because of the lack of clear information out there on the disease and the difficulty in finding medical personnel who really understand the disorder. Once I had recovered, I realized that there were many, many people suffering from the same condition who were also lost in a medical quagmire of confusing instructions, mis-diagnosis and living with a horrible disorder that destroys any real quality of living. That's what led to the idea for this book. My purpose was to help people like me – people with reactive hypoglycemia who are wading through all of the confusing information (or lack of information) on the condition. Note that I'm not calling it a "disease" here, because reactive hypoglycemia is a symptom of a disease or disorder – it isn't actually a disease in its own right. That said, sometimes you might not know what is causing your reactive hypoglycemia (the processes that regulate your blood sugar are very complex). That doesn't mean it can't be treated – usually, dietary and lifestyle changes are all that's needed to get you on the road to recovery.

In the first section of this book, you'll find a discussion of the physiology behind reactive hypoglycemia. This section also contains the causes of the disorder, which are many. You might be pre-diabetic, or you might have something more minor.

The remainder of the book walks you through the five steps you should take to combat your reactive hypoglycemia. In the vast majority of cases, the treatment for all forms of reactive hypoglycemia – whether you have pre-diabetic reactive hypoglycemia or a genetic defect – are exactly the same. That treatment consists of a fairly radical lifestyle overhaul. You'll need to look at your diet, stress levels, and other factors. It's not as easy as saying "eat six small meals a day", but it's an easy program to stick to if you take small steps. The key is to make small changes in your life over time. The freedom that comes without being chained to an emergency can of soda is worth the effort of overhauling your daily habits. You can think of the five step program – which starts with a diagnosis – as a way to break your food addictions.

This book isn't intended to give medical advice. Rather, you should use it as a complement to your physician's advice. Follow the lifestyle changed outlines in the five step program in this book, and hopefully your reactive hypoglycemia will be a distant memory.

Allison Francis

What is Reactive Hypoglycemia?

Reactive hypoglycemia is a term used to describe the hypoglycemia (low blood sugar) that occurs two to four hours after a meal. It's called "reactive" because, for the most part, your body is reacting to food. Another name for reactive hypoglycemia is postprandial hypoglycemia:

Postprandial = symptoms occur after meals (post "after" + Latin prandium "luncheon")
Hypoglycemia = low blood sugar

Simply put, reactive hypoglycemia happens like this: you consume a meal that is typically high in carbohydrates. The resulting imbalance from this carbohydrate-heavy meal is reactive hypoglycemia—low blood sugar—which causes a wide range of symptoms including sweating, shaking and mental confusion.

At first, researchers thought reactive hypoglycemia was either non-existent, a psychiatric disorder ("all in the head") or it was connected to diabetes; while diabetics suffer from not enough insulin, reactive hypoglycemics may have *too much* insulin, although this isn't always the case. A pre-diabetic who is experiencing blood sugar highs and lows will sometimes see their glucose levels rise very high (over 200 mg/dL) within a couple of hours after a meal; non-diabetics with reactive hypoglycemia may have normal highs (under 200 mg/dL) but can experience severe lows (below 40 mg/dL).

Confusing the possibility of a correct diagnosis is the fact that the low blood sugar symptoms for pre-diabetics, diabetics and non-pre-diabetics are indistinguishable. No matter what the cause of your low blood sugar, the symptoms are all the same.

Symptoms can include:

Anxiety – you might feel on edge or nervous. Some people may be prone to panic attacks.
Apathy – you don't feel like doing anything, you feel lazy, or you might feel like taking a nap at odd times – even when you are getting enough sleep.
Belligerence – low blood sugar can simply make you cranky and argumentative.

"Experts believe low levels of blood sugar may be linked to marital arguments, confrontations and even domestic violence. " (Huffington Post).

Blurred vision – although not a common symptom, low blood sugar can cause your vision to get a little hazy.

Depression – blood sugar affects the mood, usually in a negative way. Sometimes, depression, anxiety disorders and low blood sugar can go hand in hand.

Difficulty in thinking, or "brain fog."

Dizziness or faintness – you might feel like you are going to pass out.

Feeling unable to perform complex tasks, like driving or working on the computer.

Hunger – hunger pains are your body's way of telling you that your blood sugar is low and you need to eat.

Irritability -- if you often feel annoyed or irritable, blood sugar could be affecting your mood.

Lethargy – a feeling of sluggishness.

Nightmares – If you are awake with low blood sugar, it can cause anxiety. If this happens when you are asleep, the chemical changes in your brain that cause anxiety could cause nightmares instead.

Heart palpitations – a physical sign that your blood sugar is too low.

Personality changes – low blood sugar could cause a normally happy person to feel miserable, or a patient person might become impatient.

Rage – uncontrollable anger might mean that your blood sugar is too low.

Seizures -- rare in non-diabetics --blood sugar levels have to be extremely low for this to occur.

Sleeplessness – could be caused by low blood sugar levels overnight. Often this can be avoided by eating protein before bed.

Slurred speech – a sign that your brain isn't functioning correctly due to low blood sugar.

Stomach upsets – blood sugar that constantly dips and rises can cause your stomach to become queasy or upset.

Sweating -- cold sweats, usually starting on the hands and feet, are one of the classic signs of low blood sugar.

Tingling of the hands and feet – may accompany a sweating sensation.

Tremors/Shakes – sometimes comes with a feeling of anxiety.

Un-coordination (appearing drunk).

Weakness – patients often describe the weakness as flu-like or just "not feeling right."

You may have just some of the above symptoms or you may have odd symptoms that aren't listed here. The most common symptoms are cold and clammy hands, brain fog and feeling faint. However, each person is different and the confusing array of symptoms is just one reason why a diagnosis can sometimes be tough to get.

The Biology of Reactive Hypoglycemia

It's almost impossible to get a handle on your reactive hypoglycemia unless you know what is going on in your body. If you find reading about the body a bit dry, feel free to skip this chapter. You can always refer back to it later.

The two organs in the body which control blood sugar are the pancreas and the liver. The liver is a large organ weighing about 3 pounds. It is found on the right side of your upper abdomen at the bottom of your rib cage. Normally you can't feel it, because it is protected by the rib cage.

The liver works with the gallbladder, pancreas and intestines to process food, detoxify chemicals in your body and metabolize drugs. You're probably more familiar with the liver in relation to alcohol (the liver processes alcohol in the body), but the liver also works to store fuel.

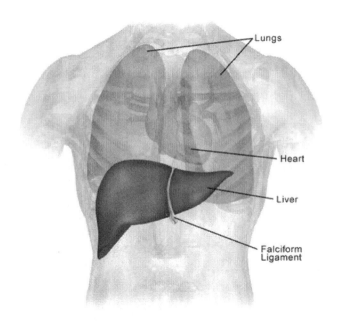

Placement of the Liver

The pancreas is nestled next to the first part of your small intestine.

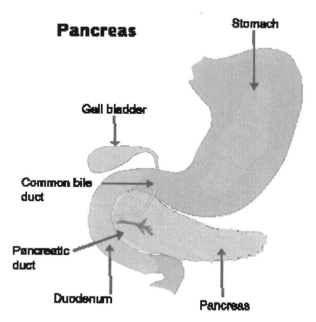

Pancreas

Stomach

Gall bladder

Common bile
duct

Pancreatic
duct

Duodenum

Pancreas

Islets are small clusters of cells in the pancreas. The islets come in three major types:

1. Alpha cells, which secrete a hormone called glucagon, one of the primary hormones that control blood sugar levels.
2. Beta cells, which secrete insulin. Insulin also plays an important role in maintaining optimal blood sugar levels.
3. Delta cells, which secrete the hormone somatostatin. Somatostatin works with insulin and glucagon to regulate the storage of glucose and control the flow of nutrients in your body.

The liver stores fuel for your body in the form of glycogen. Glycogen is released or stored depending on how high (or low) your blood glucose levels are and what hormones are being released from the pancreas.

Insulin

Insulin acts to get glucose into your cells, with the exception of the brain and the liver, which don't require insulin to uptake glucose. Insulin uses a transporter, called GLUT-4, which transports glucose into cells. Insulin also stimulates the liver to store glucose in the form of glycogen. As the primary purpose of insulin is to get fuel into your cells, it also stands to reason that insulin is responsible for decreasing levels of glucose in your bloodstream. When blood sugar concentrations fall, insulin production is halted. Diabetes is a result of too-little insulin. Without enough insulin, your cells are unable to uptake glucose, meaning that your cells don't have enough fuel although there is technically enough sugar in your body.

Glycogen

When your blood glucose is high, the liver stores the excess glucose in the liver in the form of glycogen. When blood glucose falls, this glycogen gets converted back to sugar and then released from the liver, raising your blood sugar level.

Glucagon

Glucagon is a hormone produced in the pancreas. It has the opposite effect of insulin; it increases the glucose level in the blood. When blood glucose levels dip too low, your body must pump additional glucose into the blood. Glucagon is the mechanism that signals the liver to dispense glucose into the body. It achieves it by stimulating the breakdown of glycogen stored in the liver. Glucagon can also be released by eating protein-rich meals or by exercising. However, it is not known if the exercise itself results in the secretion of glucagon or if it is the exercise-induced low blood sugar that causes the secretion.

Insulin Excess

Insulin excess is often called the *opposite of diabetes.* With diabetes, there isn't enough insulin; with insulin excess, there's too much insulin. Insulin excess can happen in two ways:

1.   A diabetic patient who injects too much insulin for their caloric intake and exercise level. This is a condition known as insulin shock.

2.   A non-diabetic individual's insulin level rises abnormally due to (rarely) a β-cell tumor or (more commonly) if their cells are over-responsive to glucose. In this second condition, the β-cells secrete more insulin than needed after a high-carbohydrate meal. The

excess insulin forces too much glucose into cells, resulting in hypoglycemia.

Reactive hypoglycemia occurs when the whole glucose regulatory system – including insulin and glucagon-- fails to work properly. It's basically where something is amiss in the regulatory system that controls how much glucose is coming in to your system, and how much is going out. This complex system can be disturbed by many things including epinephrine, insulin, glucagon, cortisol, and growth hormone imbalances.

The biology of reactive hypoglycemia is therefore complex. While "low blood sugar" *sounds* like a simple ailment to understand -- it sounds like you just need to eat something to raise your blood sugar, right? – the reality is there are a lot of complex processes involved in keeping your glucose levels stable. A disruption in these processes can be caused by dozens of different things, from eating a high-carbohydrate meal to stress. And unfortunately, even though most of the causes of reactive hypoglycemia are now known (in the next chapter, we look at some of the more common causes for reactive hypoglycemia), you may not be able to find out the reason why your blood sugar is getting out of balance. There's currently no test that can tell you how stress is affecting your blood sugar, or how much exercise you can do before your blood sugar dumps. That's why it's so important to take a multi-faceted approach to your blood sugar issues, in order to cover all of your bases.

Common Causes

At the end of the twentieth century, reactive hypoglycemia was often referred to as "idiopathic," meaning that the cause of it was not known. In many cases, the medical establishment doubted it was a disease at all. An article that appeared in *Diabetes* in 1973 (Anthony) evaluated 37 patients with reactive hypoglycemia and listed 13 as being "idiopathic." In other words, the authors did not know what was causing the reactive hypoglycemia. The authors went on further to suggest a link between reactive hypoglycemia and a personality disorder.

Hofeldt had this to say about it in 1989:

"Reactive hypoglycemia is a relatively uncommon meal-induced disorder...other disorders can be attributed as a cause for symptoms, especially neuropsychiatric disease."

In other words, it was thought for some time that the disease was "all in your head" or attributable to some kind of mental illness.

Much research has thankfully been performed in the area of reactive hypoglycemia since the 1990s. However, the notion still persists in some members of the medical establishment that reactive hypoglycemia isn't a "real" disease unless you are pre-diabetic.

Most causes are now known. Here are some of the more common causes (and a few of the rarer ones) of reactive hypoglycemia.

- Above average IQ

According to James Webb, the author of Misdiagnosis and Dual Diagnosis of Gifted Children, about six percent of highly-gifted children suffer from reactive hypoglycemia. The children who fall into this category are usually slender and exhibit intense behavior. It is thought that highly gifted, energetic children simply use up available brain fuel quickly.

- Helicobacter Pylori Infection

A common stomach bacterium can lead to reactive hypoglycemia, according to current research. If you have other symptoms such as bloating or nausea, a breath test from your doctor can rule in the presence of this bacterium.

- Insulin, Epinephrine, and Glucagon Sensitivities & Deficiencies

A 1971 study suggested that an exaggerated insulin response could be a major cause of reactive hypoglycemia. Closely related to an exaggerated insulin response is an exaggerated response of glucagon-like-peptide-1 (GLP-1), which will also cause an increase in insulin and a defect in glucagon. These types of diagnosis can only be received with lab tests.

- Alimentary hypoglycemia

If you have had gastric bypass surgery and you are experiencing reactive hypoglycemia with nausea, a feeling of fullness, weakness and heart palpitations, you could be suffering from *dumping syndrome*, where the stomach empties too fast into the small intestine. Although dietary and lifestyle changes can resolve the symptoms of dumping syndrome, some people may need medication or surgery. If you think you have dumping syndrome, make sure your health care provider is aware of your symptoms.

- Body Type

Although not a "cause" per-se, your body type can be a contributing factor. Reactive hypoglycemia often occurs in three specific types of people (although it is not limited to these people).
1. Very lean people.
2. People who have lost a lot of weight through slimming.
3. Women who are moderately overweight (not obese) in their lower body.

- Diet

Some studies indicate that a low fat, high carbohydrate diet contributes to reactive hypoglycemia. Internist Richard Podell states that 40% of his patients with sugar-related problems improve after they start an anti-hypoglycemic diet: one that is free of simple carbohydrates like white bread and pasta. These patients are also sugar, caffeine and alcohol restricted. Also, people on a calorie restricted diet may also be at risk, especially when eating primarily high-carbohydrate foods. Other factors that may contribute to the disease include alcohol (one experiment showed that the equivalent of three gin and tonics can cause reactive hypoglycemia) and there is also a possibility that a calcium deficiency in the diet may be a cause.

- Prediabetes

Typically, a prediabetic patient will not only have *hypo*glycemia but they will also have *hyper*glycemia, or high blood sugar. It's worth considering prediabetes as a possible cause for what you think is reactive hypoglycemia if you have risk factors for diabetes.

- Insulinoma

Insulinoma is a rare (4 cases per 1 million person-years) tumor of the pancreas that requires a 48 to 72 hour fasting test to diagnose. Due to the extreme rarity of this disease, if you have reactive hypoglycemia it is highly unlikely that insulinoma is the cause of your symptoms.

- Galactosemia and Hereditary Fructose Intolerance

Both galactosemia and hereditary fructose intolerance are very rare disorders. People with these diseases will typically have an enlarged liver, be jaundiced, and vomit after meals, as well as experiencing reactive hypoglycemia.

- Renal glycosuria

If increased insulin isn't present, there is a possibility of renal glycosuria, a rare disorder where glucose is excreted in the urine.

- High insulin sensitivity

Thought to be a major cause of reactive hypoglycemia, it is not thought that high insulin sensitivity by itself causes hypoglycemia, rather it works with other factors (i.e. abnormally low glucagon production) to produce reactive hypoglycemia.

- Yeast Infections

If you are reactive hypoglycemic, and sometime in the distant past you took antibiotics, it's possible you could have an overgrowth of yeast in your system. Other symptoms of a yeast overgrowth include bloating, gas and feeling queasy. Make sure you include probiotics in your diet, which can be obtained from yogurt, probiotic drinks and supplements.

- Celiac Disease / Wheat and Gluten Allergies

Many celiac patients experience hypoglycemia as a result of celiac disease. Celiac disease is an allergy to gluten, found in wheat and barley. With celiac, simple carbohydrates are absorbed through the stomach lining and more complex carbohydrates, which should be absorbed in the small intestine, aren't absorbed at all. The result is a complex pattern of apparent reactive hypoglycemia.

Like reactive hypoglycemia, celiac disease can have an array of hard to diagnose symptoms and signs:

- Abdominal cramping/bloating
- Abdominal distention
- Flatus (Passing gas)
- Gluten ataxia (a loss of balance and coordination)
- Appetite (Increased to the point of craving)
- Mouth sores or cracks in the corners
- Back pain (Such as a result of collapsed lumbar vertebrae)
- Muscle cramping (Especially in the hands and legs)
- Constipation

- Night blindness
- Decreased ability to clot blood
- Skin (Very dry and rashes)
- Dehydration
- Unusual stools (loose, frothy etc.)
- Diarrhea
- Tongue (Smooth or geographic - looks like different continents)
- Edema
- Tooth enamel defects
- Electrolyte depletion
- Weakness
- Energy loss
- Weight loss
- Fatigue

If you have reactive hypoglycemia and you haven't yet found the cause, consider celiac disease as a potential culprit, especially if you also experience any of the symptoms of celiac. For more information about celiac disease, you can visit CSA Celiacs website at www.csaceliacs.org.

There may be other causes for reactive hypoglycemia that haven't been uncovered yet. No matter what the cause though, making lifestyle changes will help to improve your symptoms. In many cases, these changes can completely eradicate your symptoms.

The Five Steps

1. Get a diagnosis
2. Eliminate these from your diet
3. Keep a journal and monitor your blood sugar
4. Tailor your diet
5. De-stress with complementary and alternative medicine techniques

One: Get a Diagnosis

Getting a diagnosis from a physician for reactive hypoglycemia is a must for many reasons, including the fact that you'll want to find out the underlying cause for your reactive hypoglycemia. A few rare, but serious conditions (like insulinoma) can't be treated with lifestyle changes. Both pre-diabetic hypoglycemia (insulin resistance) or non-diabetic reactive hypoglycemia (insulin senstitivity) or "idiopathic reactive hypoglycemia" (a nice way of saying they are unable to diagnose the cause) can all be treated by lifestyle changes.

The gold standard for diagnosis of reactive hypoglycemia is the Hyperglucidic Breakfast Test or ambulatory testing. However, if your doctor suspects your reactive hypoglycemia might be caused by pre-diabetes, he may order a 3-hour or 5-hour glucose tolerance test (GTT). However, a GTT isn't usually necessary for two main reasons:

1. The GTT is not effective as a diagnostic tool for non-diabetic reactive hypoglycemia.
2. Cheaper, faster options for diagnosing diabetes are available, such as the fasting plasma glucose test or causal plasma glucose and the A1C.

What is the Hyperglucidic Breakfast Test?

In 1995, French researcher Jean-Frédéric Brun and colleagues developed a "Hyperglucidic breakfast test" to recreate the type of meal that typically causes reactive hypoglycemia. In this test a patient is given a meal of bread, butter, and jam (a breakfast staple in Europe!) along with a serving of milk and powdered coffee, equivalent to a typical high-carbohydrate symptom-inducing meal: 9.1% protein, 27.5% fat, and 63.4% carbohydrates. After consuming this meal, your blood will be drawn at several intervals after the test.

What is Ambulatory Testing?

You can do this yourself, if you are comfortable and familiar with blood glucose monitors, or your physician may ask you to perform the test under his guidance. When symptoms occur (sweating, shakiness, palpitations etc.), you prick your finger with a special lancet, wipe a small speck of blood onto a test strip, and insert the strip into a meter. The whole process takes less than five minutes. After the machine gives you your blood glucose level, you note your blood glucose level in a food diary. A look back at your previous meal should give you an indicator of what foods may be causing your symptoms. You should also consume sugar/carbohydrates (for the purposes of this test, any high-sugar/ carbohydrates food will work: a teaspoon of honey, a few pieces of candy, a soda) after you have taken your blood sugar measurement and note if it helps with the symptoms.

A drawback with this method is that you may be feeling too sick and frustrated to get this gadget to work properly if your blood sugar is too low. A second drawback is that by the time you experience symptoms, your body may already be compensating for too much insulin, and raising your blood glucose levels; by the time you prick your finger, your blood glucose level may already be above the threshold for a reactive hypoglycemia diagnosis. Still, it remains one of the most inexpensive and reliable ways that you can find out what your blood sugar levels are looking like over time.

Oral Glucose Tolerance Test (OGTT)

Your physician may order a glucose tolerance test if they suspect diabetes, but this test is unreliable for the diagnosis of reactive hypoglycemia. If you are prone to blood sugar lows, this test can make you feel completely miserable – it can bring on all of the symptoms of reactive hypoglycemia (sweats, shakes, feeling faint etc.), but you cannot eat during the entire test.

In this test, you'll fast overnight. In the morning, a blood sample will be drawn and you'll be asked to drink a liquid with glucose. Your blood will be taken every half an hour to an hour after you drink the solution. Normal results are:

- Fasting: 60 to 100 mg/dL

- 1 hour: less than 200 mg/dL

- 2 hours: less than 140 mg/dL

If your readings are higher, this may mean you have diabetes.

The GTT is a reliable test for the detection of diabetes but returns a high number of false positives for reactive hypoglycemia. In other words, patients can experience reactive hypoglycemia on the test and not in everyday life. Some researchers (including Brun) think it should not be used as a tool to diagnose reactive hypoglycemia.

Fasting Plasma Glucose

A fasting plasma glucose test is used to confirm the presence of Type 2 diabetes. It is not used to diagnose reactive hypoglycemia. According to the American Diabetes Association, the fasting plasma glucose test is convenient, easy to do and less expensive than other tests. You'll be required to fast for 8 hours before the test. A technician will take a blood sample and send it to a lab for analysis. Usually, a diagnosis of diabetes is made if your fasting plasma glucose level is equal to or greater than 126 mg/dL on two separate tests.

A drawback to this test is that some people with pre-diabetes, some diabetics and nearly all patients with non-diabetic reactive hypoglycemia have normal fasting plasma glucose readings. Some diabetics may have normal readings which change when they eat. If your doctor suspects you might be diabetic, they may order further testing, like a GTT.

A similar blood test is the causal plasma glucose test, which is another method to diagnose diabetes (it isn't used to diagnose reactive hypoglycemia). In this simple blood test, you are not required to fast. A reading of 200 mg/dL may indicate diabetes.

A1C

The A1C test is another blood test. It's a measure of how glucose attached to hemoglobin (the protein in red blood cells that carries oxygen). Red blood cells typically survive for about three months, so this test reflects an average of your blood glucose levels for the previous three months. The test does not require fasting, so it can be performed at any time of the day. The test is usually used to help diabetics manage their condition. However, it can be used to diagnose pre-diabetes or diabetes. In 2009, the international expert committee recommended the A1C test as one of the tests available to help diagnose type 2 diabetes and prediabetes.

Results:
Normal (below 5.7 percent)
Possible diabetes (6,5 percent or over)
Pre-diabetes (5.7 to 6.4 percent)

Whipple Triad

A diagnostic tool at your doctor's disposal is something called the "Whipple Triad"; if you can answer yes to the following three questions you are most likely to be diagnosed with reactive hypoglycemia.

1. Do you have physical symptoms typical of hypoglycemia?
2. Do you also have low plasma glucose (as shown by the Hyperglucidic Breakfast Test or on ambulatory testing)?
3. Do your physical symptoms disappear when your glucose levels return to normal?

The answer to **all three** questions must be yes in order for you to get a diagnosis of reactive hypoglycemia.

Finally, make sure you ask your doctor to check you for vitamin and mineral deficiencies. Low levels of vitamins and minerals can be causing or contributing to hypoglycemic episodes. For example, low levels of calcium have been linked to reactive hypoglycemia.

Two: Eliminate these from your diet

Simple dietary changes may resolve your symptoms completely. Several studies have shown that many patients' symptoms disappear shortly after following a carbohydrate restricted diet. Most of the culprits are the processed foods in modern society, like bread and pasta. Concentrating on eating fresh, non-processed foods (including fruit, vegetables, fish, nuts, beans, dairy) can improve your symptoms. You should eliminate the following foods from your grocery list:

- Supermarket bread products: white bread, bagels, pizza, burger buns, or other "white" bread products. During the refining process, nearly all of the fiber and nutrients are lost. Substitute whole grain products instead.
- White spaghetti noodles: substitute whole grain products. Be careful to find "whole grain" and not "whole wheat."
- Most breakfast cereals. Look for basic cereals with no added sugars. These can often be found in the organic section of grocery stores or in local health food stores.
- Sugar, maple syrup and high fructose corn syrup. Use agave syrup as a replacement in moderation.
- Rice milk and soy milk that has been sweetened with sugar or high fructose corn syrup.
- Anything that has "sugar" or "high fructose corn syrup" as an ingredient. Check your labels. You might find hidden sugars in packaged meals, soups, canned beans, yogurts, ice-cream, fruit cups, and baked goods
- Sodas and fruit juices, including diet sodas. Some research has suggested that diet sodas are as bad for blood sugar control as regular soda.
- Pastries, muffins, cakes, and other "treats".
- Most restaurant meals, unless you know the protein/carb content and that it doesn't come laden with sugar.

- White potatoes, including baked potatoes and fries: except in small amounts, in a soup for example.
- Potato chips and tortilla chips.
- Fruit: eat in very small amounts with a protein like nuts or cheese.
- Coffee and alcohol. You may be able to drink these in moderation with a protein source (i.e. cheese).

What do I eat when I have a blood sugar emergency?

If you are diabetic, low blood sugar can be a medical emergency. It can also be a medical emergency if you are non-diabetic but are prone to hypoglycemic episodes that result in unconsciousness (fainting or seizures). In these cases, you should take steps to raise your blood sugar levels as soon as possible. The American Diabetes Association recommends 15 grams of simple carbohydrates:

- glucose tablets (follow package instructions)
- gel tube (follow package instructions)
- 2 tablespoons of raisins
- 4 ounces (1/2 cup) of juice or regular soda (not diet)
- 1 tablespoon sugar, honey, or corn syrup
- 8 ounces of nonfat or 1% milk
- hard candies, jellybeans, or gumdrops (see package to determine how many to consume)

If you are *not* diabetic, consuming sugar (or any form of it) will ultimately make you feel worse. Your blood sugar level will quickly return to normal. It actually might spike a little higher than normal, because you consume a 100% carbohydrate meal. Later – probably after an hour or two – your blood sugar will crash again. You should consume a carbohydrate (not sugar!) and a protein. Examples:

- Milk
- Cheese
- Yoghurt
- Nuts
- A small (4oz) cup of juice followed by a high-protein food, like fish.

Three: Keep a Journal and Monitor your Blood Sugar

If you have reactive hypoglycemia, keeping a journal and using a blood sugar monitor is a must.

Write down:

1. What you eat.
2. When you eat it.
3. When you exercise and what your readings are before and after you exercise.
4. What time of day it is when your symptoms are worst.

Basically, you are looking for further clues to try and figure out why your crashes are happening. Perhaps it's stress at work, arguing with your spouse, not getting enough sleep, or too much exercise. Any of these (and many more) could be individual triggers for you.

Although monitors tend to be on the expensive side (around $100), you can often get these for free online – you will just have to purchase testing strips and lancets from your local pharmacy. Keeping a journal and testing your blood sugar has several benefits:

1. You can track your progress. For example, when you eliminate the "bad" foods from your diet, it may take your blood sugar levels several weeks to stabilize. This could lead you to lose faith and hop back onto the cola and cookies bandwagon. If you are writing down your blood sugar levels, you should see a gradual decrease in high and low readings.

2. You can find out what other foods might be triggering your reactive hypoglycemia. For most of us, carbohydrates are the cause of reactive hypoglycemia: Specifically, meals laden with carbohydrates. However, you may have an allergy or intolerance to certain foods. Writing down what you eat, when you eat it, and what your blood sugar readings are 2

hours or so after meals will help you pinpoint any culprits.

3. Note the ratio of carbohydrates, fat and protein you are consuming. This can help you tailor your diet. For example, if you tend to have blood sugar lows after eating 25% protein with meals, you may find your symptoms don't appear after eating 30% of protein.

4. Note the time between meals. Many people with reactive hypoglycemia eat several small meals a day. However, there's no prescription about how often you *should* eat. With a proper diet, you may be able to eat 4 times a day. Or you may need to eat every 2 hours.

5. Note your current state of health. If you are ill, say with a cold or a stomach virus, this can affect how your body metabolizes food.

Four: Tailor your diet

Tailor your diet based on what you have learned from your journal. You may find you need to eat lots of small, frequent meals and snacks throughout the day. Or you may find (as I did), that you can't do any strenuous exercise for more than 20 minutes at a time without resting and eating. In addition to modifying your diet based on your journal, you may find it helpful to educate yourself about the hypoglycemic index of foods.

The Hypoglycemic Index

So you have eliminated all of the foods in the "Foods to Avoid" section. Much research has been performed over the last few decades into what types of foods spike blood sugar and which foods do not. The result is the Glycemic Index, a database of foods and how those foods affect blood glucose levels. According to the University of Sydney, the glycemic index is:

"...a ranking of carbohydrates on a scale from 0 to 100 according to the extent to which they raise blood sugar levels after eating. Foods with a high GI are those which are rapidly digested and absorbed and result in marked fluctuations in blood sugar levels. Low-GI foods, by virtue of their slow digestion and absorption, produce gradual rises in blood sugar and insulin levels, and have proven benefits for health. Low GI diets have been shown to improve both glucose and lipid levels in people with diabetes (type 1 and type 2). They have benefits for weight control because they help control appetite and delay hunger. Low GI diets also reduce insulin levels and insulin resistance."

The University of Sydney hosts the official website of the glycemic index (www.glycemicindex.com), which can help you make better choices about what foods to eat. You can search by high-glycemic foods, low-glycemic foods or a myriad of other options. You should eat high-glycemic foods in moderation – and always with a protein. Some people may not be able to tolerate some high-glycemic foods at all; that's why keeping a diary is a good idea to see how you react to different foods. The following foods are just some of the listed foods that have a high glycemic index, meaning that they will raise your glucose levels more than other foods types (a high spike can lead to a crash a couple of hours later). There are hundreds more high-glycemic foods listed on the site:

- Bananas
- Sweet corn
- Honey
- Mango
- Cherries
- Black grapes
- Kiwi
- Raisins
- Watermelon
- Peaches
- Pineapple
- White potato
- Sweet potato
- Pumpkin
- Rice (white or brown)
- Microwave popcorn
- Couscous

The following foods are some of the foods listed as low glycemic:

- Apple
- Apple juice
- Carrots
- Corn on the cob
- Milk (except for condensed milk)
- Oranges
- Pears
- Fromage Frais
- Yogurt (most types)
- Beans
- Peas
- Chickpeas
- Lentils
- Soy beans
- Nuts
- Egg fettuccini
- Eggs

There are hundreds more low-glycemic foods listed. The site also lists the glycemic index of meals which allows you to combine higher-glycemic foods with lower ones to make a low-glycemic meal. For example, vegetarian or meat lasagna and White rice (Oryza sativa), boiled, eaten with fish, tomato and onion sauce are both low-glycemic meals.

A good idea would be to *only* eat foods that are low on the index, and then – over time – introduce higher-glycemic foods slowly back into your diet to see which you can tolerate.

Although the next section offers some suggested recipes, a thorough description of the glycemic index and a suggested diet plan using the glycemic index is beyond the scope of this book. We recommend the following books if you are interested in reading more:

The G.I. Diet: The Easy, Healthy Way to Permanent Weight Loss by Gallop, Rick and Sole M.D., Michael J.

The Glycemic-Load Diet: A powerful new program for losing weight and reversing insulin resistance by Thompson, Rob

500 Low Glycemic Index Recipes: Fight Diabetes and Heart Disease, Lose Weight and Have Optimum Energy with Recipes... by Logue, Dick

Recipe Suggestions

Dinners & Lunches

Glazed Mahi Mahi

4 servings

3 Tbsp agave nectar
3 Tbsp Bragg's liquid aminos
3 Tbsp balsamic vinegar
1 tsp grated fresh ginger root
1 clove garlic crushed or to taste 2 tsp olive oil
4 (6 oz) mahi mahi fillets
 salt and pepper to taste
1 Tbsp vegetable oil

Procedure

1. In a shallow glass dish, stir together the agave, Bragg's, balsamic vinegar, ginger, garlic and olive oil. Season fish fillets with salt and pepper, and place them into the dish. If the fillets have skin on them, place them skin side down. Cover, and refrigerate for 20 minutes to marinate.
2. Heat vegetable oil in a large skillet over medium-high heat. Remove fish from the dish, and reserve marinade. Fry fish for 4 to 6 minutes on each side, turning once, until fish flakes easily with a fork. Remove fillets to a serving platter and keep warm.
3. Pour reserved marinade into the skillet, and heat over medium heat until the mixture reduces to a glaze consistently.

4. Spoon glaze over fish, and serve immediately.

Preparation Time: 5 minutes
Cooking Time: 12 minutes
Total Time: 37 minutes
Nutrition Facts
Serving size: 1/4 of a recipe (10.8 ounces).
Calories:355.43
Calories from fat:74.82
Carbs:16.38g
Protein: 50.98g

Grilled Salmon

6 servings

1 1/2 pound salmon fillets
lemon pepper to taste
garlic powder to taste
salt to taste
1/3 cup Bragg's liquid aminos
1/3 cup agave nectar
1/3 cup water
1/4 cup olive oil

Procedure
1. Season salmon fillets with lemon pepper, garlic powder, and salt.
2. In a small bowl, stir together Bragg's, agave, water, and oil. Place fish in a large resealable plastic bag with the sauce mixture, seal, and turn to coat. Refrigerate for at least 2 hours.
3. Preheat grill for medium heat.
4. Lightly oil grill grate. Place salmon on the preheated grill, and discard marinade. Cook salmon for 6 to 8 minutes per side, or until the fish flakes easily with a fork.

Preparation Time: 15 minutes
Cooking Time: 16 minutes
Total Time: 2 hours

Nutrition Facts
Serving size: 1/6 of a recipe (5.7 ounces).
Calories:268.58
Calories from fat:124.60
Carbs:13.58g
Protein: 21.56g

Tuna Teriyaki

4 servings

2 Tbsp Bragg's liquid aminos
1 Tbsp Chinese rice wine
1 large clove garlic minced
1 Tbsp minced fresh ginger root 4 (6 oz) tuna
steaks (about 3/4 inch thick)
1 Tbsp olive oil

Procedure

1. In a shallow dish, stir together Bragg's, rice wine, garlic, and ginger. Place tuna in the marinade, and turn to coat. Cover, and refrigerate for at least 30 minutes.
2. Preheat grill for medium-high heat.
3. Remove tuna from marinade, and discard remaining liquid. Brush both sides of steaks with oil.
4. Cook tuna for approximately for 3 to 6 minutes per side, or to desired doneness.

Preparation Time: 15 minutes
Cooking Time: 12 minutes
Total Time: 57 minutes
Nutrition Facts
Serving size: 1/4 of a recipe (3.6 ounces).
Calories:163.67
Calories from fat:68.7
Carbs:1.91g
Protein:20.44g

Lemony Orange Roughy

4 servings

1 Tbsp olive oil
4 (4 oz) fillets orange roughy
1 orange, juiced 1 lemon, juiced
1/2 tsp lemon pepper

Procedure
   1. Heat oil in a large skillet over medium-high heat. Arrange fillets in the skillet, and drizzle with orange juice and lemon juice. Sprinkle with lemon pepper. Cook for 5 minutes, or until fish is easily flaked with a fork.

Preparation Time: 15 minutes
Cooking Time: 5 minutes
Total Time: 20 minutes
Nutrition Facts
Serving size: 1/4 of a recipe (4.4 ounces).
Calories:107.36
Calories from fat:35.84
Carbs:3.26g
Protein:15.14g

Basil Grilled Shrimp

6 servings

3 cloves garlic minced
1/3 cup olive oil
1/4 cup tomato sauce
2 Tbsp red wine vinegar 2 Tbsp chopped fresh basil
1/2 tsp salt
1/4 tsp cayenne pepper
2 pounds fresh shrimp, peeled and deveined
Wooden skewers

Procedure

2. In a large bowl, stir together the garlic, olive oil, tomato sauce, and red wine vinegar. Season with basil, salt, and cayenne pepper. Add shrimp to the bowl, and stir until evenly coated. Cover, and refrigerate for 30 minutes to 1 hour, stirring once or twice.
3. Preheat grill for medium heat. Thread shrimp onto skewers, piercing once near the tail and once near the head. Discard marinade.
4. Lightly oil grill grate. Cook shrimp on preheated grill for 2 to 3 minutes per side, or until opaque.

Preparation Time: 15 minutes
Cooking Time: 6 minutes
Total Time: 55 minutes

Nutrition Facts
Serving size: 1/6 of a recipe (6.4 ounces).
Calories:222.69
Calories from fat:120.59
Carbs:
Protein:21.16g

Tuna Salad

4 servings

Ingredients
1 (7 ounce) can white tuna, drained and flaked
6 tablespoons mayonnaise or salad dressing
1 tablespoon Parmesan cheese
3 tablespoons sweet pickle relish
1/8 teaspoon dried minced onion flakes
1/4 teaspoon curry powder
1 tablespoon dried parsley
1 teaspoon dried dill weed
1 pinch garlic powder

Procedure

1. In a medium bowl, stir together the tuna, mayonnaise, Parmesan cheese, and onion flakes.
2. Season with curry powder, parsley, dill and garlic powder.
3. Mix well and serve with crackers or on a sandwich.

Prep: 10 mins
Cook:
Ready: 10 mins

Nutrition:
Calories 228 kcal
Carbohydrates 5.3 g
Fat 17.3 g

Protein 13.4 g
Tuna Salad with Egg
2 servings

Ingredients
1 (6 ounce) can chunk light tuna, drained
1/4 cup creamy salad dressing (such as Miracle Whip®)
1 hard-boiled egg, chopped
1/2 apple, diced
1/2 cup chopped toasted pecans
salt and pepper to taste

Procedure
1. Stir the tuna, salad dressing, egg, apple, and pecans together in a bowl; season with salt and pepper.
2. Chill in refrigerator at least 1 hour before serving.

Prep: 10 mins
Cook:
Ready: 1 hr 10 mins

Nutrition:
Calories 432 kcal
Carbohydrates 12.8 g
Fat 31 g
Protein 27.2 g

Mock Tuna Salad
2 servings

Ingredients
1 (19 ounce) can garbanzo beans (chickpeas), drained and mashed
2 tablespoons mayonnaise
2 teaspoons spicy brown mustard
1 tablespoon sweet pickle relish
2 green onions, chopped
salt and pepper to taste

Procedure
1. In a medium bowl, combine garbanzo beans, mayonnaise, mustard, relish, chopped green onions, salt and pepper.
2. Mix well.

Prep: 20 mins
Cook:
Ready: 20 mins

Nutrition:
Calories 220 kcal
Carbohydrates 32.7 g
Fat 7.2 g
Protein 7 g

Gourmet Egg Salad Sandwich

4 servings

Ingredients

4 slices bacon
4 hard-cooked eggs, chopped
1/4 cup mayonnaise
1 teaspoon yellow mustard
salt and ground black pepper to taste
4 slices sourdough bread
2 tablespoons pesto
4 slices Jarlsberg cheese

Procedure

1. Place bacon in a large skillet and cook over medium-high heat, turning occasionally, until evenly browned, about 10 minutes. Drain bacon slices on paper towels; crumble.
2. Preheat oven broiler and set rack about 6 inches from heat source.
3. Mix eggs, mayonnaise, mustard, salt, and pepper in a bowl; fold in crumbled bacon.
4. Toast sourdough bread under broiler until lightly browned, about 2 minutes. Spread pesto evenly on each slice of bread; top with 1/4 egg salad mixture and spread to cover completely. Top each sandwich with 1 slice Jarlsberg cheese.

5. Return sandwiches to broiler and cook until cheese is melted, 2 to 3 minutes. Served sandwiches warm and open-faced.

Prep: 5 mins
Cook: 15 mins
Ready: 20 mins

Nutrition:
Calories 445 kcal
Carbohydrates 17.3 g
Fat 31.9 g
Protein 21.8 g

Black Bean Veggie Burgers
4 servings

Ingredients
1 (16 ounce) can black beans, drained and
rinsed
1/2 green bell pepper, cut into 2 inch pieces
1/2 onion, cut into wedges
3 cloves garlic, peeled
1 egg
1 tablespoon chili powder
1 tablespoon cumin
1 teaspoon Thai chili sauce or hot sauce
1/2 cup bread crumbs

Procedure
1. If grilling, preheat an outdoor grill for high heat, and lightly oil a sheet of aluminum foil. If baking, preheat oven to 375 degrees F (190 degrees C), and lightly oil a baking sheet.
2. In a medium bowl, mash black beans with a fork until thick and pasty.
3. In a food processor, finely chop bell pepper, onion, and garlic. Then stir into mashed beans.
4. In a small bowl, stir together egg, chili powder, cumin, and chili sauce.
5. Stir the egg mixture into the mashed beans. Mix in bread crumbs until the

mixture is sticky and holds together. Divide mixture into four patties.
6. If grilling, place patties on foil, and grill about 8 minutes on each side. If baking, place patties on baking sheet, and bake about 10 minutes on each side.

Prep: 15 mins
Cook: 20 mins
Ready: 35 mins

Nutrition:
Calories 198 kcal
Carbohydrates 33.1 g
Fat 3 g
Protein 11.2 g

General Tao's Chikin

4 servings

1 package Quorn chick'n chunks OR 1lb chicken, cut into chunks
1 egg
3/4 cup cornstarch
4 Tbs sesame oil
3 chopped green onions
1 Tbsp minced ginger
1 Tbsp minced garlic
2/3 cup vegetable stock
2 Tbsp soy sauce
3 Tbsp fructose
 red pepper to taste
1 Tbsp sherry, optional
1 Tbsp cornstarch dissolved in 2 tablespoons water
1 Tbsp white vinegar

Procedure

1. Whisk egg in a small bowl. Empty Quorn into the bowl and toss to coat.
2. Sprinkle 3/4 cup cornstarch over Quorn, toss to coat (do not overtoss).
3. Fry Quorn for 8 minutes, medium high heat in a wok. Push to one side.
4. Add green onions, ginger, garlic to the wok center, cook for 2 minutes.
5. Add vegetable stock, soy sauce, fructose, red pepper and vinegar.

6. Add cornstarch to the center and heat thoroughly until bubbling.
7. Push the Quorn to the center and mix well.

Nutrition Facts
Serving size: ¼ recipe
Calories: 515.36
Calories from fat: 182.24
Carbs: 55.97g
Protein: 25.9g

Indian Stuffed Peppers
4 servings

The slow cooker will do all of the work for you in this dish. All you have to do for dinner is slice the tops from the peppers, remove the seeds, fill with the filling, and bake.

4 large red bell peppers
1 cup chopped onion
2 tsp yellow mustard
1 tsp cumin seeds
1 tsp ground coriander
½ tsp salt
¼ tsp cayenne pepper
2 cups shredded green cabbage
1 cup diced sweet potato
2 cups cooked chickpeas
1 Tbsp minced fresh ginger
3 cloves garlic, minced (about 1 Tbs.)
¼ cup vegetable broth
¼ cup chopped cilantro
2 Tbsp chopped roasted cashews
3/4 cup plain yogurt
2 ½ Tbsp prepared mango chutney

Procedure
1. Place onion, yellow mustard, cumin seeds, coriander, salt, cayenne pepper, cabbage, potato, chickpeas, ginger, garlic, and vegetable broth in a slow cooker. Cook for 6 hours.

2. When done, stir in cilantro and cashews.
3. Slice tops off peppers and remove seeds. Fill with slow cooker filling and place caps on top.
4. Place peppers in a deep baking pan. Place ½" water in the pan and cover with foil.
5. Bake for 40 minutes at 375 degrees.
6. Combine yogurt and chutney. Drizzle over peppers to serve.

Nutrition Facts
Serving size: ¼ recipe
Calories: 337.31
Calories from fat: 48.8
Carbs: 58.27g
Protein: 13.04g

Jamaican Jerk Chili

8 servings

1 can kidney beans, drained and rinsed
1 can red beans, drained and rinsed
1 can diced tomatoes, 14.5oz
1 can tomato purée, 14.5oz
4 ea red potatoes cut into bite-sized pieces
1 pkg vegetarian meat crumbles 8oz OR 12 oz ground beef
1 large onion, chopped
2 Tbsp vinegar
2 Tbsp jerk seasoning (check for sugar content)
½ cup water
1 Tbsp fructose
¼-½ tsp minced Scotch bonnet or habanero chile, or to taste

Procedure

1. Combine all ingredients in 4-qt. slow cooker.
2. Stir in ½ cup water. Cook for 6-8 hours on low. Yield: 8

Nutrition Facts
Calories: 219.18
Calories from fat: 10.61
Carbs: 42.16g
Protein: 11.75g

Kidney Bean Burger
6 servings

Use Ezekiel 4:9 buns for this burger (available in health food stores), and serve with a garden salad.

2 cans kidney beans, drained and rinsed well
1 onion
2 cloves garlic
3/4 cup whole wheat bread crumbs
1/8 cup whole wheat flour
1 Tbsp tomato paste
1 Tbsp cayenne pepper
1 ea egg
½ tsp oregano
½ tsp salt
1 spray olive oil

Procedure
1. Chop garlic and onion in a food processor. Add everything else and process until blended. Divide into 6 balls. Flatten into ½" patties.
2. Spray a frying pan with olive oil.
3. Cook on medium 4-5 minutes each side.

Nutrition Facts
Calories: 219.58
Calories from fat: 15.98
Carbs: 40.73g
Protein: 11.3g

Egg and Hash Brown Pie
8 servings

6 strips Morningstar veggie bacon, chopped
5 eggs
1/2 cup milk 3 cups hash brown potatoes, thawed
1/3 chopped green onions
1 1/2 cup shredded cheddar cheese, divided

Procedure
1. Place veggie bacon in a large, deep skillet. Cook over medium high heat until evenly brown. Crumble, and set aside.
2. Preheat oven to 350 degrees F (175 degrees C). Lightly grease a 7x11 inch baking dish.
3. In a large bowl, beat together the eggs and milk. Stir in the bacon, hash browns, green onions, and 1 cup shredded Cheddar cheese. Pour into the prepared baking dish.
4. Bake in the preheated oven 25 to 35 minutes, or until a knife inserted in the center comes out clean. Sprinkle the remaining Cheddar cheese on top, and continue baking for 3 to 4 minutes, or until the cheese is melted. Remove from oven, and let sit 5 minutes before serving.

Preparation Time: 15 minutes
Cooking Time: 45 minutes
Total Time: 1 hour and 5 minutes
Nutrition Facts

Calories:244
Calories from fat:124.06
Carbs:16.96g
Protein: 12.83g

Irish Eggs

4 servings

2 Tbsp olive oil
2 large potatoes peeled and diced into 1/4"
chunks
1 onion minced
1/2 teaspoon turmeric 1 teaspoon chili powder
1 green bell pepper, chopped
6 eggs beaten

Procedure

1. In a large skillet, warm olive oil over medium low heat. Add potatoes, onion and green pepper. Cover pan; sauté until potatoes are browned. Stir frequently.
2. Add turmeric and chili powder. Stir well.
3. Push potatoes to one side of pan. Add eggs to pan and then scramble until done. Mix with potatoes and serve.

Yield: 4
Preparation Time: 15 minutes
Cooking Time: 20 minutes
Total Time: 35 minutes
Nutrition Facts
Serving size: 1/4 of a recipe (8.6 ounces).
Calories:255.09
Calories from fat:188.97
Carbs:22.33g
Protein:12.28g

Breakfast Burritos

6 servings

12-16 oz extra firm tofu, drained, pressed and crumbled OR 12 oz lean ground beef
1 ea small yellow onion, peeled and diced
2 ea garlic cloves, minced or pressed
1 ea bell pepper, diced
2 ea small red potatoes
4 Tbsp olive oil
½ tsp turmeric
1 pinch salt
1 pinch pepper
6 tortillas
½ cup mushrooms, quartered or sliced (optional)
1 ea jalapeno, sliced
1 cup red, yellow peppers, diced
2 ea breakfast sausage patties, diced
½ cup cheese, grated
6 Tbsp fresh salsa

Procedure
1. Preheat oven to 375º Fahrenheit.
2. Chop the potatoes into bite sized pieces. Place in a Ziplock bag with 1T olive oil and a dash of salt and pepper.
3. Bake potatoes for 20 minutes.
4. While waiting for potatoes to cook, heat 3T olive oil in a frying pan.

5. Add garlic and vegetables. Cook on medium heat until the onions are softened.
6. Add tofu and turmeric.
7. Add sausage. Cook for 5 minutes, stirring occasionally until sausage is heated through.
8. Place warm tortilla on a plate. Fill with 1/6 of the tofu mixture and 1T of salsa.
9. Divide the cheese between the burritos. Roll up and enjoy!

Nutrition Facts
Calories: 355.93
Calories from Fat: 156.63
Carbs: 38.58g
Protein:12.07g

Breakfast Scramble
4 servings

For the sauce:
½ cup flour
½ cup nutritional yeast
1 tsp garlic powder
2 cups water
1 tsp yellow mustard
4 tbsp or less margarine
For the stir fry:
½ onion
4 strips bacon OR veggie bacon
½ green pepper
6 ea eggs, free range
3 Tbs olive oil
 Salt and pepper, to taste

Procedure
1. Mix flour, nutritional yeast, garlic powder, and water in a small saucepan. Heat on medium until thick and bubbling.
2. Remove from heat. Add mustard and margarine.
3. Sauté onion and green pepper in 1T olive oil for 3-4 minutes until soft.
4. Add 2T more oil.
5. Add whisked eggs.

6. While eggs are cooking, microwave bacon until crispy (add 30 seconds to the suggested package timing).
7. Sauté this for another couple of minutes.
8. Add salt and pepper to taste.
9. Add crumbled bacon, salt and pepper, and sauce from small saucepan. Sauté for 2 minutes and serve.

Nutrition Facts
Calories:159.28
Calories from Fat: 91.64
Carbs:14.77g
Protein:2.11g

Lemon Baked Cod

4 servings

Ingredients
1 lb cod fillets
1/4 cup butter, melted
2 tablespoons fresh-squeezed lemon juice
1/4 cup rice flour
1/2 teaspoon salt
1/8 teaspoon white pepper
paprika
Parsley sprigs and lemon wedges for garnish

Procedure
1. Cut fillets into serving size pieces.
2. Mix the butter and lemon juice.
3. Mix flour, salt and white pepper in a separate bowl.
4. Dip fish into butter mixture and then coat with the flour mixture.
5. Place fish in an ungreased 8" square baking pan.
6. Pour remaining butter mixture over fish and then sprinkle with paprika.
7. Cook uncovered in 350 degree oven until fish flakes easily with fork, 25-30 minutes. Garnish with parsley sprigs and lemon slices if desired.

Prep: 10 mins
Cook: 25 mins
Ready: 35 mins

Nutrition:
Calories 225.2
Carbohydrates 6.5 g
Fat 12.3 g
Protein 21.2 g

Dijon Baked Cod

4 servings

1/4 cup mayonnaise
2 teaspoons Dijon mustard
2 teaspoons horseradish (jarred)
1 tablespoon fresh-squeezed lemon juice
1/8 cup breadcrumbs
1 tablespoon parmesan cheese
4 (6 ounce) cod fillets
1 tablespoon butter
1/4 cup breadcrumbs
1 tablespoon parmesan cheese

Procedure

1. Preheat oven to 350°F and lightly grease a baking sheet.
2. Mix mayonnaise, mustard, horseradish and lemon juice in a small bowl; stir in parmesan cheese and 1/8 cup of bread crumbs.
3. Arrange fish portions on prepared cooking sheet, spread mixture evenly over fish.
4. Mix melted butter, bread crumbs and 1 tablespoon parmesan cheese in a bowl. Sprinkle over the cod.
5. Bake for 15-20 minutes until cod flakes easily with a fork.

Prep: 5 mins
Cook: 15 mins
Ready:20 mins

Nutrition:
Calories 283.5
Carbohydrates 11.5 g
Fat 10.3 g
Protein 34.4 g

Chili, Cumin and Lime Cod

2 - 4 servings

2 lbs fresh cod fillets
1 teaspoon chili powder
1/2 teaspoon fresh chopped cilantro
1/2 teaspoon salt
2 tablespoons butter
1/4 teaspoon cumin
1 lime, juiced

Procedure
1. Preheat oven to 450°F.
2. Coat a baking dish with cooking spray. Place cod in pan.
3. Sprinkle chili powder and salt over fish.
4. Roast 5-7 minutes until opaque and fish flakes easily with a fork.
5. Melt butter in small saucepan.
6. Add cilantro, cumin and lime juice and cook for 1 more minute.
7. Before serving drizzle butter mixture over cod.

Prep: 10 mins
Cook: 7 mins
Ready: 17 mins
Nutrition:
Calories 485.6
Carbohydrates 2.8 g
Fat 14.8 g
Protein 81.4 g

Crabmeat Stuffed Haddock

6 servings

Ingredients
3 tablespoons olive oil
1 stalk celery, finely chopped
3 green onions, finely chopped
1 teaspoon minced garlic
1(6 ounce) can lump crabmeat, drained
3 slices dry white bread, crusts removed and cubed
1/4 teaspoon salt
1/4 teaspoon ground black pepper
1 egg, beaten
1/2 cup grated Romano cheese
2 tablespoons lemon juice
1 tomato, seeded and diced
1/8 teaspoon ground black pepper
5 tablespoons butter, melted
6 (4 ounce) haddock fillets
Toothpicks

Procedure

1. Preheat oven to 375 degrees F. Lightly grease a 9x13 inch baking dish.
2. Heat olive oil in a heavy skillet over medium heat for 2-3 minutes. Add celery, green onion and garlic.
3. Stir fry for 3-4 minutes until soft. Remove from heat, and stir in the crabmeat, bread cubes, egg, Romano

cheese, lemon juice, and tomato. Season with salt and 1/4 teaspoon of pepper. Mix until well blended.

4. Lay the haddock fillets in the prepared baking dish. Brush with melted butter. Place a generous tablespoon of the crab mixture onto half of each fillet, and fold the other half over to cover. Secure with toothpicks. Sprinkle on any remaining stuffing, and drizzle with any leftover melted butter. Cover the dish with aluminum foil.

5. Bake for 20 minutes. Remove the cover and bake for an additional 10 minutes, until the top has browned and the fish flakes easily with a fork.

Prep: 15mins
Cook: 40 mins
Ready: 55 mins
Nutrition:
Calories 365 kcal
Carbohydrates 9 g
Fat 21.5 g
Protein 32.9 g

Seafood a la Creole

6 servings

3/4 teaspoon dried oregano
1/2 teaspoon salt
1/2 teaspoon ground white pepper
1/2 teaspoon ground black pepper
1/2 teaspoon cayenne pepper
1/2 teaspoon fresh thyme, chopped
1/2 teaspoon fresh sweet basil
1/4 cup butter
1 cup peeled and chopped tomato
3/4 cup chopped onion
3/4 cup chopped celery
3/4 cup chopped green bell pepper
1 1/2 teaspoons minced garlic
1 1/4 cups fish stock
1 cup canned tomato sauce
1 teaspoon agave nectar
1/2 teaspoon hot pepper sauce (I like Chalula)
2 bay leaves
1 pound peeled and deveined shrimp
1 pound bay scallops
1 pound haddock fillets cut into bite-sized pieces

Procedure
1. Mix the oregano, salt, white pepper, black pepper, cayenne pepper, thyme, and basil in a small bowl.

2. Melt butter in a large skillet over medium heat; stir in tomato, onion, celery, green bell pepper, and garlic. Stir-fry until the onion is translucent, about 5 minutes.
3. Stir in fish stock, tomato sauce, agave, hot pepper sauce, and bay leaves. Reduce heat to low and bring sauce to a simmer. Stir in seasoning mix and simmer until the flavors have blended, about 20 minutes.
4. Gently stir in shrimp, bay scallops, and haddock; bring sauce back to a simmer and cook until the shellfish and fish are opaque, about 20 more minutes. Remove bay leaves to serve.

Prep: 30 mins
Cook: 40 mins
Ready: in 1 hr 10 mins
Nutrition:
Calories 328 kcal
Carbohydrates 11.8 g
Fat 10 g
Protein 47.2 g

Breakfast

Scrambled Eggs
1 serving

Ingredients
2 eggs
1 teaspoon mayonnaise or salad dressing
1 teaspoon water (optional)
1 teaspoon margarine or butter
salt and pepper to taste (optional)

Procedure
1. In a cup or small bowl, whisk together the eggs, mayonnaise and water using a fork.
2. Melt margarine in a skillet over low heat. Pour in the eggs, and stir constantly as they cook.
3. Remove the eggs to a plate when they are set, but still moist. Do not overcook. Never add salt or pepper until eggs are on plate, but these are also good without.

Prep: 2 mins
Cook: 4 mins
Ready: 6 mins

Nutrition:
Calories 210 kcal
Carbohydrates 1 g
Fat 17.4 g
Protein 12.7 g

Hard Boiled Egg

8 eggs

1 tablespoon salt
1/4 cup distilled white vinegar
6 cups water
8 eggs

Procedure

1. Combine the salt, vinegar, and water in a large pot, and bring to a boil over high heat. Add the eggs one at a time, being careful not to crack them. Reduce the heat to a gentle boil, and cook for 14 minutes.
2. Once the eggs have cooked, remove them from the hot water, and place into a container of ice water or cold, running water.
3. Cool completely, about 15 minutes.
4. Store in the refrigerator up to 1 week.

Prep: 5 mins
Cook: 20 mins
Ready: 40 mins

Nutrition:
Calories 72 kcal
Carbohydrates 0.4 g
Fat 5 g
Protein 6.3 g

Oven Scrambled Eggs
12 servings

1/2 cup butter or margarine, melted
24 eggs
2 1/4 teaspoons salt
2 1/2 cups milk

Procedure
1. Preheat the oven to 350 degrees F (175 degrees C).
2. Pour melted butter into a glass 9x13 inch baking dish. In a large bowl, whisk together eggs and salt until well blended. Gradually whisk in milk. Pour egg mixture into the baking dish.
3. Bake uncovered for 10 minutes, then stir, and bake an additional 10 to 15 minutes, or until eggs are set. Serve immediately.

Prep: 10 mins
Cook: 25 mins
Ready: 35 mins

Nutrition:
Calories 236 kcal
Carbohydrates 3.2 g
Fat 18.6 g
Protein 14.3 g

Baked Omelet Roll

6 servings

6 eggs
1 cup milk
1/2 cup all-purpose flour
1/2 teaspoon salt
1/4 teaspoon ground black pepper
1 cup shredded Cheddar cheese

Procedure

1. Preheat oven to 450 degrees F (230 degrees C).
2. Lightly grease a 9x13 inch baking pan.
3. In a blender, combine eggs, milk, flour, salt and pepper; cover and process until smooth. Pour into prepared baking pan.
4. Bake in preheated oven until set, about 20 minutes. Sprinkle with cheese.
5. Carefully loosen edges of omelet from pan. Starting from the short edge of the pan, carefully roll up omelet. Place omelet seam side down on a serving plate and cut into 6 equal sized pieces.

Prep: 5 mins
Cook: 20 mins
Ready: 25 mins
Nutrition:
Calories 206 kcal
Carbohydrates 10.5 g
Fat 12.1 g
Protein 13.4 g

Baby Spinach Omelet

1 serving

Ingredients
2 eggs
1 cup torn baby spinach leaves
1 1/2 tablespoons grated Parmesan cheese
1/4 teaspoon onion powder
1/8 teaspoon ground nutmeg
salt and pepper to taste

Procedure

1. In a bowl, beat the eggs, and stir in the baby spinach and Parmesan cheese. Season with onion powder, nutmeg, salt, and pepper.
2. In a small skillet coated with cooking spray over medium heat, cook the egg mixture about 3 minutes, until partially set.
3. Flip with a spatula, and continue cooking 2 to 3 minutes.
4. Reduce heat to low, and continue cooking 2 to 3 minutes, or to desired doneness.

Prep: 6 mins
Cook: 9 mins
Ready: 15 mins
Nutrition:
Calories 186 kcal
Carbohydrates 2.8 g
Fat 12.3 g
Protein 16.4 g

Five: De-stress with Complementary Medicine

According to Dr. Lawrence Wilson, if your body is placed under any kind of stress at all, it can result in reactive hypoglycemia. "Stress" can include exercise, hunger or simply an emergency. When you get stressed, your body reacts by burning fuel faster to compensate for all of the stress hormones that are flooding your body. Your goal is to avoid anything that will cause your body to burn fuel fast; A dramatic drop in blood sugar will lead to a dramatic rise and an endless yo-yo of ups and downs.

"I'm going to say that I used to be a typical Type A – a stress monster. Since taking up yoga and meditation, I can't even fathom what I was thinking! Not only am I calmer overall and I'm more able to deal with simple stresses (like someone cutting me off in traffic), my reactive hypoglycemia has also improved dramatically. I did make dietary changes, but I am convinced meditation especially is a major part of that positive change." Elsie, Grand Junction CO.

Yoga

Yoga is a mind-body practice in complementary and alternative medicine (CAM) with origins in ancient Indian philosophy. The various styles of yoga that people use for health purposes typically combine physical postures, breathing techniques, and meditation or relaxation. It is not fully known what changes occur in the body during yoga; whether they influence health; and if so, how. There is, however, growing evidence to suggest that yoga works to enhance stress-coping mechanisms and mind-body awareness. Research is under way to find out more about yoga's effects, and the diseases and conditions for which it may be most helpful.

Yoga in its full form combines physical postures, breathing exercises, meditation, and a distinct philosophy. Yoga is intended to increase relaxation and balance the mind, body, and the spirit.

Research suggests that yoga might:

- Improve mood and sense of well-being.

- Counteract stress.

- Reduce heart rate and blood pressure.

- Increase lung capacity.

- Improve muscle relaxation and body composition.

- Help with conditions such as anxiety, depression, and insomnia.

- Improve overall physical fitness, strength, and flexibility.

- Positively affect levels of certain brain or blood chemicals.

Yoga is generally considered to be safe in healthy people when practiced appropriately. Studies have found it to be well tolerated, with few side effects.

- People with certain medical conditions should not use some yoga practices. For example, if you also have a disc disease of the spine, extremely high or low blood pressure, glaucoma, retinal detachment, fragile or atherosclerotic arteries, a risk of blood clots, ear problems, severe osteoporosis, or cervical spondylitis should avoid some inverted poses.

Training, Licensing, and Certification

There are many training programs for yoga teachers throughout the country. These programs range from a few days to more than 2 years.

Standards for teacher training and certification differ depending on the style of yoga.

There are organizations that register yoga teachers and training programs that have complied with minimum educational standards. For example, one nonprofit group requires at least 200 hours of training, with a specified number of hours in areas including techniques, teaching methodology, anatomy, physiology, and philosophy. However, there are currently no official or well-accepted licensing requirements for yoga teachers in the United States.

If You Are Thinking About Yoga

- Do not use yoga as a replacement for conventional care or to postpone seeing a doctor.
- Consult with your health care provider before starting yoga.
- Ask about the physical demands of the type of yoga in which you are interested, as well as the training and experience of the yoga teacher you are considering.
- Tell your health care providers about any complementary and alternative practices you use. Give them a full picture of what you do to manage your health. This will help ensure coordinated and safe care.

Meditation

There are many types of meditation, most of which originated in ancient religious and spiritual traditions. Generally, a person who is meditating uses certain techniques, such as a specific posture, focused attention, and an open attitude toward distractions. Meditation may be practiced for many reasons, such as to increase calmness and physical relaxation, to improve psychological balance, to cope with pain, or to enhance overall health and well-being.

It is not fully known what changes occur in the body during meditation; whether they influence health; and, if so, how. Research is under way to find out more about meditation's effects, how it works, and diseases and conditions for which it may be most helpful.

The term *meditation* refers to a group of techniques, such as mantra meditation, relaxation response, mindfulness meditation, and Zen Buddhist meditation. Most meditative techniques started in Eastern religious or spiritual traditions. These techniques have been used by many different cultures throughout the world for thousands of years. Today, many people use meditation outside of its traditional religious or cultural settings, for health and well-being.

In meditation, you learn to focus your attention. Some forms of meditation instruct the practitioner to become mindful of thoughts, feelings, and sensations and to observe them in a nonjudgmental way. This practice is believed to result in a state of greater calmness and physical relaxation, and psychological balance. Practicing meditation can change how you relate to the flow of emotions and thoughts.

Most types of meditation have four elements in common:

- A quiet location. Meditation is usually practiced in a quiet place with as few distractions as possible. This can be particularly helpful for beginners.
- A specific, comfortable posture. Depending on the type being practiced, meditation can be done while sitting, lying down, standing, walking, or in other positions.
- A focus of attention. Focusing one's attention is usually a part of meditation. For example, the meditator may focus on a mantra (a specially chosen word or set of words), an object, or the sensations of the breath. Some forms of meditation involve paying attention to whatever is the dominant content of consciousness.
- An open attitude. Having an open attitude during meditation means letting distractions come and go naturally without judging them. When the attention goes to distracting or wandering thoughts, they are not suppressed; instead, the meditator gently brings attention back to the focus. In

some types of meditation, the meditator learns to "observe" thoughts and emotions while meditating.

Meditation used as CAM is a type of mind-body medicine. Generally, mind-body medicine focuses on:

• The interactions among the brain/mind, the rest of the body, and behavior.

• The ways in which emotional, mental, social, spiritual, and behavioral factors can directly affect health.

Examples of Meditation Practices

Mindfulness meditation and Transcendental Meditation (also known as TM) are two common forms of meditation. NCCAM-sponsored research projects are studying both types of meditation.

Mindfulness meditation is an essential component of Buddhism. In one common form of mindfulness meditation, the meditator is taught to bring attention to the sensation of the flow of the breath in and out of the body. The meditator learns to focus attention on what is being experienced, without reacting to or judging it. This is seen as helping the meditator learn to experience thoughts and emotions in normal daily life with greater balance and acceptance.

The TM technique is derived from Hindu traditions. It uses a mantra (a word, sound, or phrase repeated silently) to prevent distracting thoughts from entering the mind. The goal of TM is to achieve a state of relaxed awareness.

How Meditation Might Work

Practicing meditation has been shown to induce some changes in the body. By learning more about what goes on in the body during meditation, researchers hope to be able to identify diseases or conditions for which meditation might be useful.

Some types of meditation might work by affecting the autonomic (involuntary) nervous system. This system regulates many organs and muscles, controlling functions such as heartbeat, sweating, breathing, and digestion. It has two major parts:

- The sympathetic nervous system helps mobilize the body for action. When a person is under stress, it produces the "fight-or-flight response": the heart rate and breathing rate go up and blood vessels narrow (restricting the flow of blood).
- The parasympathetic nervous system causes the heart rate and breathing rate to slow down, the blood vessels to dilate (improving blood flow), and the flow of digestive juices increases.

It is thought that some types of meditation might work by reducing activity in the sympathetic nervous system and increasing activity in the parasympathetic nervous system.

In one area of research, scientists are using sophisticated tools to determine whether meditation is associated with significant changes in brain function. A number of researchers believe that these changes account for many of meditation's effects.

It is also possible that practicing meditation may work by improving the mind's ability to pay attention. Since attention is involved in performing everyday tasks and regulating mood, meditation might lead to other benefits.

A 2007 NCCAM-funded review of the scientific literature found some evidence suggesting that meditation is associated with potentially beneficial health effects. However, the overall evidence was inconclusive. The reviewers concluded that future research needs to be more rigorous before firm conclusions can be drawn.

Meditation is considered to be safe for healthy people. There have been rare reports that meditation could cause or worsen symptoms in people who have certain psychiatric problems, but this question has not been fully researched. People with physical limitations may not be able to participate in certain meditative practices involving physical movement. You should speak with your health care provider prior to starting a meditative practice and make your meditation instructor aware of your condition.

If You Are Thinking About Using Meditation Practices

- Do not use meditation as a replacement for conventional care for your reactive hypoglycemia or as a reason to postpone seeing a doctor.
- Ask about the training and experience of the meditation instructor you are considering.

Acupuncture

Acupuncture may help with relaxation. Acupuncture is a family of procedures that involve stimulating anatomical points on your body using a variety of techniques. In most cases, acupuncture normally means that your skin will be penetrated with thin, solid, metallic needles that are manipulated by a practitioner's hands or by electrical stimulation. Acupuncture is a key component of *traditional Chinese medicine*, but it is also widely practiced in the United States. According to the 2007 National Health Interview Survey, which included a comprehensive survey of complementary and alternative medicine use by Americans, an estimated 3.1 million U.S. adults and 150,000 children had used acupuncture in the previous year.

- Acupuncture is a very safe procedure that is regulated by The U.S. Food and Drug Administration (FDA). For example, the FDA requires that any needles used in the procedure are sterile, nontoxic, and labeled for single use by qualified practitioners.

- If you decide to try acupuncture, make sure to check any practitioner's credentials. Most states require acupuncturists to be licensed (see the Resources section at the back of this book for information on state licensing).

Internet Resources

Articles on everything Reactive Hypoglycemia, diet, causes, website reviews, reactive hypoglycemia store, and more.
http://www.reactivehypoglycemia.info

Basic info about Reactive Hypoglycemia from the Mayo clinic. A good resource to direct friends and relatives to for a quick overview.
http://www.mayoclinic.com/health/reactive-hypoglycemia/AN00934

Basic info on Dumping Syndrome from the Mayo Clinic
http://www.mayoclinic.com/health/dumping-syndrome/DS00715/

Pathophysiology of the Digestive System.
Everything you ever wanted to know about what happens to the food you eat!!
http://arbl.cvmbs.colostate.edu/hbooks/pathphys/digestion/index.html

Overview of reactive hypoglycemia.
Article can be a bit confusing, because it interchanges the words "reactive hypoglycemia" and "hypoglycemia" but nonetheless has some good information.
http://emedicine.medscape.com/article/122122-overview

University of Dusseldorf website.
If you can get past the awkward language, this website has some interesting facts, including explaining the prediabetes-reactive hypoglycemic possible link.
http://www.uni-duesseldorf.de/MedFak/insulinoma/english%20homepage/mainpage/subpage/Epostpran_hypo.htm#top

Jean-Frédéric Brun's Website
This researcher specializes in exercise, fuel metabolism assessment in vivo, and hemorheology.

You will find an excellent academic paper here about postrprandial reactive hypoglycemia and its causes.
http://jeanfrederic.brun.free.fr/postprandial%20hypo%20review%20diabetes%20metab.pdf

The article on H-Pylori's effect on producing reactive hypoglycemia can be found online.
http://www.springerlink.com/content/j231l47rx4n611j2/

Everything you ever wanted to know about the Glycemic Index.
http://www.glycemicindex.com/

Hypoglycemia Homepage Holland.
Full of general information on reactive hypoglycemia.
http://www.hypoglykemie.nl/

Personal Story on Panic Disorder and hypoglycemia.
http://www.hastingspress.co.uk/hypo/

Sample Menu for Reactive Hypoglycemia
http://www.dialadietitian.org/nutritionpage.asp?id=1391

Eating Guidelines for Reactive Hypoglycemia
http://www.dialadietitian.org/nutritionpage.asp?id=1280

Use of Guar Gum to Prevent Alcohol Induced Reactive Hypoglycemia

http://alcalc.oxfordjournals.org/cgi/content/abstract/16/3/135

Info on the "gin and tonic" effect on reactive hypoglycemia. Full article is available with a free subscription.

CBS News Story: "Diabetes Sufferers: Beware of Caffeine"
http://www.cbsnews.com/stories/2008/01/29/health/webmd/main3763964.shtml

Armenian website with information on a variety of different causes for reactive hypoglycemia, including gastroectomy and alcohol-induced reactive hypoglycemia.

http://www.health.am/db/more/postprandial-hypoglycemia-reactive-hypoglycemia/

Nearly all of the articles and journals are available through your local library through interlibrary loan. Ask your local public library about it.

References

Liver photo: BruceBlauds|Wikimedia Commons

Açbay O,et. al.. Helicobacter pylori-induced gastritis may contribute to occurrence of postprandial symptomatic hypoglycemia.. Dig Dis Sci. 1999 Sep;44(9):1837-42.

Airola, P. Hypoglycemia: A better approach. Phoenix, Arizona: Health Plus Publishers, 1977.

American Diabetes Association. Standards of medical care in diabetes--2013. *Diabetes Care*. 2013 Jan;36 Suppl 1:S11-66.

Anthony, B.A. et.al Personality Disorder and Reactive Hypoglycemia: A Quantitative Study doi: 10.2337/diab.22.9.664Diabetes September 1973vol. 22 no. 9 664-675

Baumel, S. Dealing with depression naturally. Lincolnwood Illinois: Keats Publishing. 2000

Brun JF, Fédou C, Bouix O, Raynaud E, Orsetti A. Evaluation of a standardized hyperglucidic breakfast test in postprandial reactive hypoglycaemia. Diabetologia, 1995, 38, 494-501.

Brun JF, Fedou C, Mercier J. Postprandial Reactive Hypoglycemia. Diabetes Metab. 2000 Nov;26(5):337-51.

Buse JB, Polonsky KS, Burant CF. Type 2 diabetes mellitus. In: Melmed S, Polonsky KS, Larsen PR, Kronenberg HM, Larsen PR, eds. *Williams Textbook of Endocrinology*. 12th ed. Philadelphia, Pa.: Elsevier Saunders; 2011:chap 31.

Buss RW, Kawsal PC, Roddam RF. Mixed meal tolerance test and reactive hypoglycemia. Horm Metab Res, 1982, 14, 281-283.

Chalew SA, Mc Laughlin JV, Mersey JH, Adams AJ, Cornblath M, Kowarski A. The use of the plasma epinephrine response in the diagnosis of idiopathic postprandial syndrome. JAMA, 1984, 251,612-615.

Charles MA, Hofeldt F, Shackelford A. Comparison of oral glucose tolerance tests and mixed meals in patients with apparent idiopathic post-absorptive hypoglycemia. Diabetes, 1981, 30, 465-470.

Chen M, Bergman RN, Porte D Jr. Insulin resistance and b-cell dysfunction in aging: the importance of dietary carbohydrate. J Clin Endocrinol Metab, 1988, 67, 951-957.

Christensen, L. et. al. Dietary alteration of somatic symptoms and regional brain electrical activity. Biological Psychiatry. 29 (7). 1991. Pp. 679-682

Cryer PE, Binder C, Bolli GB, Cherrington AD, Gale EAM, Gerich JE, Sherwin RS. Hypoglycemia in IDDM. Diabetes, 1989, 38, 1193-1199.

Donaldson, David. Psychiatric Disorders With a Chemical Basic. Informa Health Care, 1998

Duyff, R.American Dietetic Association complete food and nutrition guide. Hoboken, NJ: Wiley & Sons. 2006.

Fabrykant M, Pacella BL. The association of spontaneous hypoglycemia with hypocalcemia and electro-cerebral dysfunction. Proc Am Diab Assoc, 1947, 7, 233-236

Goodpaster BH, Kelley DE, Wing RR, Meier A, Thaete FL. Effects of weight loss on regional fat distribution and insulin sensitivity in obesity. Diabetes, 1999, 48, 839-847.

Harris S. Hyperinsulinism and dysinsulinism. J Amer Med Ass, 1924, 83, 729-733.

Harris,P. et. al. Endocrinology in clinical practice. London: Martin Dunitz Ltd. 2003. p.475 and Lippincott Williams and Wilkins, Professional Guide to Diseases. 2009.

Heinrich Heine University of Dusseldorf. Article posted on website University of Dusseldorf. Retirved May 18 2009 from http://www.uni-duesseldorf.de/MedFak/insulinoma/english%20home page/mainpage/subpage/Epostpran_hypo.htm#top

Hofeldt FD. Reactive hypoglycemia. Metabolism, 1975, 24, 1193-1208.

Hofeldt. FD. Reactive Hypoglycemia. Endocrinol Metab Clin North Am. 1989 Mar;18(1):185-201.

Huffington Post. Keep Arguing With Your Spouse? Hunger And Low Blood Sugar Could Be To Blame... PA/The Huffington Post UK | Posted: 15/04/2014

Inzucchi SE, Sherwin RS. Type 2 diabetes mellitus. In: Goldman L, Schafer AI, eds. *Goldman's Cecil Medicine*. 24th ed. Philadelphia, Pa.: Elsevier Saunders; 2011:chap 237.

Johnson DD, Door KE, Swenson WM, Service FJ. Reactive hypoglycemia.JAMA, 1980, 243, 1151-1155.

Lefèbvre PJ, Andreani D., Marks V, Creutzfeld W. Statement on postprandial a or reactive a hypoglycaemia (Letter). Diabetes Care, 1988, 11, 439.

Lefèbvre PJ. Heurs et malheurs de l'hyperglycémie provoquée par voie orale. In: Journées Annuelles de Diabétologie de l'Hôtel-Dieu, 1987. Flammarion Médecine-Sciences, Paris, 313-322

Lefebvre PJ. Hypoglycemia or non-hypoglycemia. In: Rifkin H, Colwell JA, Taylor SI (eds) Diabetes 1991. Proceedings of the 14th International Diabetes Federation Congress, Washington DC, June 1991.

Excerpta Medica Amsterdam London New York Tokyo, 1991, 757-761.

Lefèbvre PJ. Hypoglycemia: post-prandial or reactive. Current therapy in Endocrinology and Metabolism, 1988, 3, 339-341, and Lefèbvre PJ. Hypoglycemia or non-hypoglycemia. Acta Clinica Belgica,

Letiexhe MR, Scheen AJ, Gérard PL, Desaive C, Lefèbvre PJ. Insulin secretion, clearance and action before and after gastroplasty in severely obese subjects. Int J Obes Relat Metab Disord, 1994, 18, 295-300

Lev-Ran A, Anderson RW. The diagnosis of postprandial Hypoglycemia. Diabetes, 1981, 30, 996-999

Luyckx AS, Lefèbvre PJ. Plasma insulin in reactive hypoglycemia. Diabetes, 1971, 20, 435-442.

Malaisse, W. et. al. Effects of Artificial Sweeteners on Insulin Release and Cationic Fluxes in Rat Pancreatic Islets. Laboratory of Experimental Medicine, Brussels Free University, 808 Route de Lennik, B-1070 Brussels, Belgium

Mirouze J, Pham TC, Selam JL, Bringer J, Chenon D. Posthyperglycaemic hypoglycaemia: effects of somatostatin. Nouv Presse Med, 1981, 10, 2947-2949.

O'Keefe SJD, Marks V. Lunchtime gin and tonic: a cause of reactive hypoglycaemia. Lancet, 1977, i, 1286-1288.

Owada K, et.al. Highly increased insulin secretion in a patient with postprandial hypoglycemia: role of glucagon-like peptide-1 (7-36) amide. Endocr J, 1995, 42, 147-151.

Pfeiffer, C. Mental and Elemental Nutrients: a physician's guide to nutrition and health care. New Canaan, CT: Keats Publishing, 1975.

Raghavan, A. Srinivasan, V. & Snow, K. Hypoglycemia. Medscape.com. Retrieved May 15 2009 from http://emedicine.medscape.com/article/122122-overview

Raine, A. (1993). The psychopathology of crime: Criminal behavior as a clinical disorder. San Diego, CA: Academic Press.

Raynaud E, Perez Martin A, Brun JF, Fedou C, Mercier J. Insulin sensitivity measured with the minimal model is higher in moderately overweight women with predominantly lower body fat. Horm Metab Res, 1999, 31, 415-417.

Service JF. Hypoglycemic disorders. N Engl J Med, 1995, 332,1144-1152.

Stein,J. Internal Medicine. St. Louis, Missouri: Mosby, Inc, 1998.

The American Diabetes Association. Hypoglycemia (low blood glucose). http://www.diabetes.org/living-with-diabetes/treatment-and-care/blood-glucose-control/hypoglycemia-low-blood.html#sthash.0WcmlHor.dpuf

The International Expert Committee. International Expert Committee report on the role of the A1C assay in the diagnosis of diabetes. *Diabetes Care*. 2009;32(7):1327–1334.

Wilson, Lawrence MD. Hypoglycemia. http://drlwilson.com/articles/HYPOGLYCEMIA.htm

Yamamoto T, Oya Y, Furusawa Y, Nonaka I, Murata M. Successful treatment of recurrent hypoglycemia by pioglitazone in a patient with myotonic dystrophy]

[Article in Japanese]Rinsho Shinkeigaku. 2009
Oct;49(10):641-5.[

Zonera Ashraf Ali, MD, and Klaus Radebold, MD, PhD.
Retrieved May 15 2009 from:
http://emedicine.medscape.com/article/283039-
overview